# THE ABCS (AND FS) OF STRENGTH TRAINING

## A SIMPLIFIED SYSTEM TO ASSESS JUST ABOUT EVERYTHING

**Dan John**

Paperback: 978-1-963675-08-5

Published by OS Press

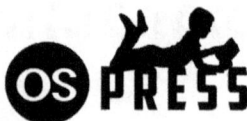

# Contents

Thank you to Tim Anderson and all his friends in the Original Strength community for making this very easy for me.

Thank you to the OS Press team for REALLY making life easy as a wandering writer.

Thank you to all my athletes who sweated and strained through the F workouts that we don't dare discuss.

## Important Note

Exercise has risks associated with it. Research shows it can lead to being stronger, healthier, and happier. However, it can also lead to injuries or even death. It happens.

You should also know that doing nothing also has risks associated with it. Research shows that being sedentary can lead to sickness, weakness, frailty, depression, and anxiety. It can also make you more injury-prone and hasten your destination towards death. It happens.

Consult your trusted family physician before beginning any exercise program or engaging in any sedentary lifestyle.

My daughter, Kelly, gets on me because I judge everything. In truth, I only judge squat depth. Actually, she is right: I judge everything. I might judge a lot, but I have a system for it. It's based on cost-to-benefit ratios, also known as "risk to rewards." Let me explain how I do this method.

I've been using this chart for a long time. This is a picture that I took from one of my workshops.

My Mental Exercise and "Go To" Decision Matrix:

# The Biggest Bang for the Buck!

### Cost to Benefit Ratios

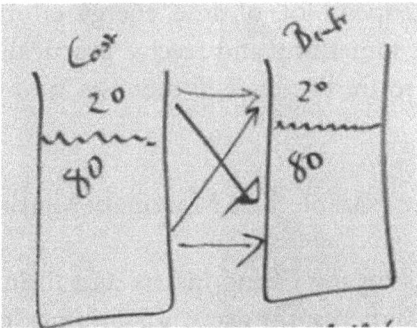

### Pareto's Law...the Two Test Tubes

A: 20% of your effort, your investments, your work, your time gives you 80% of your Benefits. (O lifts, Royalties)

B: 80% in/80% back (We EXPECT this) (Powerlifts/Job/Fiber)

C: 20% in/20% back ("Acres of Diamonds")

F: 80% in/20% back (Stop!!! Doing this!)

But, WE THRIVE on Errors.

To make this idea work, we must learn to judge things a bit. Getting a college education is certainly a long-term benefit, but if you have millions of dollars in student debt, the costs need to be discussed. So, I like to use my brain a bit, "judge" things, and assign grades. (Before you ask, I have no "D" grades!)

> A: Low cost in terms of time, money, equipment, and effort. Weirdly high return. These are the gems of life.

B. Reasonable costs, reasonable returns. You basically get what you put in, and the benefits take care of you. I usually use fiber in food as my first example because, first, it is funny to say, and, second, most people understand this at the gut level (and that's funny, too).

C. Low entry costs and "you get what you get." For me, it's a local workshop (I've taken them on fermenting foods, time management, personal growth, writing, poetry, and fitness) that cost little and each time, I came away with a few ideas. Often, it can be me saying "yes" to a business idea and testing it out. It can also be a new exercise or training concept. As Earl Nightingale taught us, these are the Acres of Diamonds at your feet. You never know which will translate to something huge (an A Grade).

F. These are the worst. If you spend lots of time, energy, effort, money, and brain power on something and receive practically nothing in return, run! There are F friends, F exercises, and F decisions. Stop!

Let's add some detail with my favorite example: The Movement Matrix.

You can see some of the "A" grades on my lifting matrix and lifting programs. These are life's jewels. With my throwers, 15 minutes of Olympic lifts gives them the most (maybe all) they need from the weight room. Royalties are wonderful checks that I get from work I did well over a decade ago (in some cases). These have low costs and massive benefits. There are also plenty of "B" grades. Here it is.

# The Movement Matrix
## EACH is "Key!" Each is an A or a B

| Movement | Planks as a Program | Strength Training (Less than 10 reps) / Hypertrophy (15-25 reps) | Anti-Rotation Work | Triads | Olympic Lifts |
|---|---|---|---|---|---|
| Push | PUPPs<br>Plank | (Bench) Press<br>Push-up | 1 Arm Bench Press<br>1 Arm Overhead Press | Push press/jerk | |
| Pull | TRX Rows<br>Bat Wing<br>Ts and Ys | Pull-up<br>Row | 1 arm TRX Row | | Squat Snatch |
| Hinge | Gluteal Bridge with AB Hold | Hip Thrust<br>Rack DLs<br>Goat Bag Swing | Hill Sprints/<br>Stadium Steps<br>Skipping/Bounding/<br>High Knee Work | Swing | |
| Squat | Goblet Squats<br>6 point Rocks | Dbl KB Front Squat<br>The Whole Squat Family | Bear Hug Carries<br>Bear Crawls<br>Bear Hug Carries with Monster Walk | Litvisprints, Litvisleds | Clean & Jerk |
| Loaded Carry | Farmer's Walk<br>Horn Walk | Prowler<br>Car push | 1 arm carries:<br>Suitcase Carry<br>Waiter Walk<br>Rack Walk | | |

Before we look closely at the matrix, if you think about it, you probably have "A" friends, too. The other day, I was on the phone with my old training partner, Eric. We always pick up right where we left off last time. It's always positive, always fun. We don't burden each other when we converse. It's always great. In business and life, I love my "A" relationships.

For food, protein and water get top marks. Regarding general exercise, I'm not sure you can find anything better than walking in terms of the cost-to-benefit ratio. These get top marks!

B grades are things that you get what you put into it. Fiber is the obvious choice, but it's the 9-5 job and the basic lifts. I don't necessarily love Marvel movies, but you know, walking in the door, you are going to "get this kind of entertainment." The bulk of the barbell world would represent the B grades for me. You get the benefits from the work you put in.

The best business advice I ever received was to have a barbell strategy. Simply, keep (or get) that 9-5 job that provides income, insurance, benefits, and stability. On the other end of the barbell, you keep that dream (in my case, writing about lifting) alive in your spare moments. Soon, if you are on the right path, the 9-5 job is surpassed by the hobby! This is the value of the Bs: they give you amazing benefits and keep you in a place where you can find the As. Or, in my case, **grow the As.**

Remember this: I will try something new and different very soon. I don't know what exercise, lift, diet idea, or recovery tool I will use, but I will spend time, treasure, and talent trying to make it work. This new idea might be a total waste of effort, or it might transform everything I do. These little experiments, the C grades, keep me returning to learn more and seek the next A.

**Grow the As.**

C grades are those little adventures where you meet somebody or accept a small job. With some exercises, like hip thrusts, I saw them as a "yeah, I will try this," and they swiftly shifted to an A grade. I will often watch a movie on a plane or a quiet evening and think, "Well, that was good." I usually never watch the show again, but the time was worth it. I'm thinking Nomadland, The Railway Man (an underappreciated Colin Firth movie), or Living (Bill Nighy in a simple film about living). I would probably include Past Lives here, too. Great movies... but I might never watch again.

So, that is the key to Cs. It's a person, thing, or whatever, that seems interesting, and maybe it is so amazing that it slides over to the A category. Many of my training movements started as little experiments that spilled over into the A category.

But many other short experiments were just that: short experiments. I learned a lesson or two and walked away. They were worth the time and energy, but I might not share them with my clients or athletes. This is fine, of course.

THE ABCS (AND FS) OF STRENGTH TRAINING

And, of course, if it does make the A grade, you know what I am going to say:

## Grow the As.

Now, the Acres of Diamonds story. I have heard many versions…usually from Earl Nightingale. I like this one:

### Dr Russell Conwell made this story famous.

*There was a man, Al Hafed, who lived on the banks of the River Indus and had a nice farm with orchards and gardens, excess cash, a beautiful wife, and children. He was 'wealthy because he was contented.' Then, an old priest visited him and, one night, related how the world was made, including the formation of all the rocks, the earth, and the precious metals and stones. He told the farmer that if he had a few diamonds, he could have not just one farm but many. The farmer listened. Suddenly, he wasn't happy with what he had thus far acquired.*

*He sold up and traveled in search of diamonds across Persia, Palestine, and Europe. A couple of years later, his money was gone, and he wandered around in rags. When a large wave came in from the sea, he was happily swept under by it.*

*The man who had bought the farmer's land was another story. One day, watering his animals in the stream that ran through the property, he noticed a glint in the watery sands. It was a diamond. In fact, it was one of the richest diamond finds in history; the mines of Golconda would yield not just one or two but acres of diamonds.*
https://www.butler-bowdon.com/russell-h-conwell---acres-of-diamonds.html

This story reminds me that the obvious first place to look is almost universally right at my feet. When someone I trust or love tells me to try something…I do it. Sometimes, those little hints end up changing my life.

And now, the Fs.

If you find yourself listening on the phone to someone, once again, bemoaning their life for hours and sucking out your life energy... again, pause for a moment and think when this same person asked anything about you, your day, or your dog. If the answer is "never," you might have an F friend. I have a pretty good idea of what I consider F exercises, F diets (not the F-Plan Diet, which is actually pretty good), and F decisions.

Stop F-ing around and get rid of Fs!

And...**grow the As.**

# The Movement Matrix

| Movement | Planks as a Program | Strength Training (Less than 10 reps) / Hypertrophy (15-25 reps) | Anti-Rotation Work | Triads | Olympic Lifts |
|---|---|---|---|---|---|
| **Push** | **PUPPs** Plank | (Bench) Press Push-up | 1 Arm Bench Press 1 Arm Overhead Press | Push press/jerk | |
| **Pull** | **TRX Rows** Bat Wing Ts and Ys | Pull-up Row | 1 arm TRX Row | | |
| **Hinge** | **Gluteal Bridge with AB Hold** | Hip Thrust Rack DLs Goat Bag Swing | **Hill Sprints/ Stadium Steps** Skipping/Bounding/ High Knee Work | Swing | Squat Snatch / Clean & Jerk |
| **Squat** | **Goblet Squats** 6 point Rocks | Dbl KB Front Squat The Whole Squat Family | **Bear Hug Carries** Bear Crawls Bear Hug Carries with Monster Walk | Litvisprints, Litvisleds | |
| **Loaded Carry** | **Farmer's Walk** Horn Walk | Prowler Car push | 1 arm carries: **Suitcase Carry** Walter Walk Rack Walk | | |

First, the basics. The rows represent how I summarize the fundamental human movements we can work on in the weight room. I often note, "YES, we can add more movements," but I suggest you don't. People have commented that we can add horizontal and vertical to the push and pull, but not a single American athlete I have ever trained needed more upper body work vis-à-vis the lower body.

Yes, you can add a host of other things, but most of them would not be As and Bs. Trust me, I tried.

The columns represent more than just lifts or speed of movement. The planks can be seen as Isometrics, but some involve bracing your whole body while moving. That's why I call the goblet squat and farmer walk "moving planks." The next column would be recognizable as what most consider the world of weightlifting. The next column is something I struggled with understanding for decades. We don't need rotation in the weight room; we need to train anti-rotation. The Triads are combination moves that involve multiple fundamental movements (three!), and our last columns are the Olympic lifts that involve every muscle and basic movement.

It might seem complicated, but it is weirdly simple once you start using it.

A few notes: the movements in **BOLD** are exercises that can be done without any weight equipment. With some rope or straps and just some heavy stuff, a person with a good imagination can construct a fantastic training program.

One of the hardest lessons of being a strength coach is that sometimes the weights (barbells, kettlebells, dumbbells, machines, and anything else that pops into your mind) can get in the way of improvement and performance.

I will not be explaining any of the specific exercises as I explain them in articles and videos online. It's hard to explain in words when a video explains things far easier. There is one abbreviation: PUPPs. It's simple: it's the Push Up Position Plank.

As Tim Anderson of Original Strength reminds me often, this matrix goes together with Pressing RESET like "Peas and Carrots." Be sure to say this in your Forrest Gump voice. Here is how I use the matrix with OS in a complementary way:

| Movement | Planks as a Program | Original Strength Performance Resets |
|---|---|---|
| Push | PUPPs<br>Plank | Prone Neck Work<br>Bird Dog Family |
| Pull | Bat Wing | Prone Neck Work<br>Elbow Rolls |
| Hinge | Gluteal Bridge with AB Hold | Six Point Nods and Rocks<br>Bird Dog Family |
| Squat | Goblet Squats<br>6 point Rocks | Prone Neck Work<br>Hip Flexor Stretch/Rolling |
| Loaded Carry | Farmer's Walk<br>Horn Walk | Crawling and<br>CrossCrawls |

One could have an amazing life and athletic career just doing the matrix. Let me add one additional thing that will completely change one's vision of training beyond just more reps and sets.

## Level Changes

I'm not sure I have a humble opinion about anything, but I humbly think the biggest gaps in training are instantly apparent in real-world application. Something is lacking in so many programs, but once you see it, like those illusions that pop out when you finally see the trophy or dog or whatever, it becomes hard not to see it.

Generally, the two biggest gaps in training are authentic squatting (not accordion squatting, as I call it) and any and all loaded carries.

In real life, a good example is during an extended hiking trip—both of these gaps will become obvious at the first potty break. And, if you haven't been doing loaded carries, you'll pay a high price ascending the Himalayas…or helping your friends move.

Adding goblet squats and farmer walks have been game-changing additions for many of the people I work with professionally.

Do them!

Yet, people often miss another more subtle issue: the lack of levels. I'm not calling out Curves or Nautilus, but an entire workout sitting down (and seat-belted in) doesn't reflect the demands of most of life. Sitting down is one level.

"Level" is the word I use to describe the ground, half-kneeling, full-kneeling, lunge position, fully erect, and moving away in various directions. Think of the levels in the earth's crust (as a geography minor in college, I occasionally like to flex my knowledge of the planet).

Some movements, like the Turkish getup, involve almost all the levels up and down. Combining a waiter's walk at the top position moves us at virtually all levels. And, as good as TGUs are, these are not dynamic enough for every purpose.

That's why I like combining movements in a training session. We've been using lift-n-sprints for decades, and the results on the field of play have been amazing. Basically, pick a hinge or squat variation, do about 10, drop the load, and INSTANTLY sprint away. Vary the load and distance every time, but not the intensity. There's only one coaching cue: Go, go, go!!!

Hooking a sled up also works (lift-n-sleds) if you're smart enough not to put the load in the sled's path. Watching when people don't listen to the warning of keeping the load from the sled's path is funny.

Note: on the Matrix, I use the terms Litvinovs and Litvisleds instead of lift-n-sprints and lift-n-sleds.

As great as these are, many of us train in smaller spaces that don't work for "lift-n-X." This combination works wonders for the body (a special thank you to Mitchell Cook for dreaming this up):

Eight goblet squats
Prowler push (as appropriate, but 20–40 meters is great)
Eight pushups

You'll feel the hit from getting up and down off the ground and the changes in levels. Up to five rounds of this workout is appropriate, but strive for less at first. My best is 20 loops: 160 goblet squats, 160 push-ups, and 400 meters with the prowler. I was tired.

If you don't have the space to prowl, sled, or sprint, the swing, goblet squat, and pushup combination works well here. Just refer to my workout, the Humane Burpee (thank you, Dan Martin, for the name).

So, here you go:
15 Swings
5 Goblet Squats
5 Push-Ups

15 Swings
4 Goblet Squats
4 Push-Ups

15 Swings
3 Goblet Squats
3 Push-Ups

15 Swings
2 Goblet Squats
2 Push-Ups

15 Swings
1 Goblet Squat
1 Push-Up

That's 75 swings, 15 squats, and 15 pushes, which is enough to get "things done" for most people.

Mixing barbell deadlifts with bear crawls is a wonderful preseason prep workout for American football.

Once you begin to embrace training the levels, your eyes will quickly pick up the total lack of this kind of training for most people. It raises the heart rate, adds work capacity, and reflects the real world of sport and life.

Get leveled.

## Incorporating Level Changes and Groundwork into Training

I've been striving to share the idea of level changes in the weight room for a while. I have no issues with gyms that have their clients seated and training throughout a workout. This is the appropriate approach for all kinds of issues, most of which I'm not qualified to address.

Training an elderly person recovering from a total joint replacement differs from prepping a college athlete for a season. I understand that.

More is needed for the people I train. One simple idea is to take the basic movements and list the various levels we use in a typical setting.

I subcategorize the movements into three terms I learned from a student of Martha Graham, arguably one of the inventors of modern dance, who taught dance in the summer sessions while I was at Utah State. Yes, I took dance classes in the summer.

She mentioned three concepts to explore in every position and every movement:

Earth
Human
Sky

I heard this concept and instantly went to training:

> **Earth**: Look! There's the ground, and these dance courses demand a lot of time there.
> **Human**: When I heard this, I thought of jumping up and climbing trees.
> **Sky**: I was already summing all sports and lifting as "stay tall." It's human nature to get up, stand up, look around, wander… and keep looking towards the stars.

In workshops, I teach the three groups with these positions:

Earth
> On your back
> Prone (face down)
> Six points (hands, knees, and feet on the ground)
> Bear (hands and feet on the ground)
> Half-kneeling (one knee down kneeling)

Human
> Air (jumping, leaping, bounding)
> Hang
> Brachiate (think monkey bars or rope climbing)

Sky
> Squat
> Hinge
> Gait (walking, running, sprinting)
> Carry

I don't want to exhaust all the options completely, but here are some examples of level changes and fundamental human movements.

## Push...with Level Changes

"Earth"
On your Back
    Floor Press
    Turkish Get Down Press
Prone
    Push Ups and Variations
Six Point
    Arm Bends (Remedial)
Bear
    Bear Crawls/Push Ups/B Boy
Half Kneeling
    Presses (Maybe my favorite)

"Sky" (Stay Tall)
Squat
    Thrusters...Done Well
Hinge
    Clean and Press
    John McKean's GM/Dip
Gait
    Walking See-Saw Press
Carry
    Strongman Press Walk

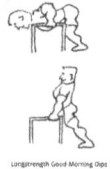

Longstrength Good-Morning Dips

## Pull...with Level Changes

"Earth"
On your Back
    Horizontal Rows
Half Kneeling
    Chops/Paddles/Rows
Hang
    By itself...Money!!!
    Pull Ups et al
Brachiate
    Monkey Bars and Javelin

"Sky" (Stay Tall)
Squat
    John McKean's Squat/Pulls
Hinge
    Rows!
    *Done Correctly*

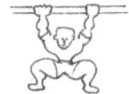

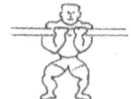

Longstrength Squat Pulls

# Hinges...with Level Changes

**"Earth"**

On your Back
    Glute Bridge/Hip Thrust
Prone
    The "Pump" (Cobra+D Dog)
Half Kneeling
    Oddly, as a complement
**"Human"**
Air
    Appropriate Jumping
    Appropriate Bounding/Skipping

**"Sky" (Stay Tall)**

Squat
    O lifts...full versions
Hinge
    KB Swings and Snatches
    Deadlifts
Gait
    Hill Sprints
    Stadium Steps
Carry
    Drags between legs

# Squat...with Level Changes

**"Earth"**

On your Back
    Brazilian Get Back Up Test
Prone
    Lower Body Rolls
Six Point
    Rocks
Bear
    Crawls
**"Human"**
Air
    Squat (GS) Jumps

**"Sky" (Stay Tall)**

Squat
    Six Point Rocks
    Assisted Squats
    Goblet Squats
    Overhead Squats
    Front/Back Squats
Carries
    Bear Hug Carries

# Loaded Carries...With Level Changes

**"Earth"**
Bear Crawls with Sleds
Half Kneeling (*Some* loaded lunges)


**"Human"**
Brachiate

**"Sky" (Stay Tall)**
Squat
    Bear Hug Carry with Squats
    Lift 'n' Sprints (Squats)
Hinge
    Lift 'n' Sprints (DLs/O lifts)
Gait
    Heavy Hands/Rucking
Carry
    The Whole Family

## Career Changer: *Loaded Carries!* Building Appropriate Work Capacity

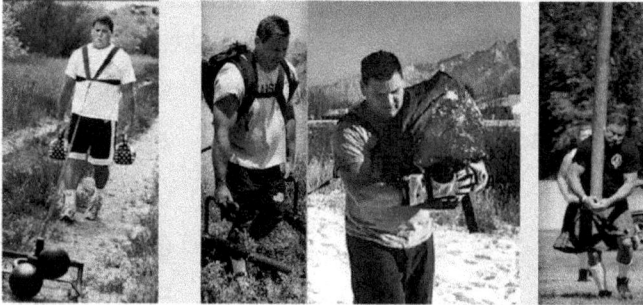

As I review the list, I see the same complaint I voice when I see most programs: There are lots of push options but fewer of the other movements. I did my best.

During the early days of the pandemic, I was asked for a one-kettlebell workout. Without thinking about level changes, I sent this idea:

> Half-kneeling press
> Hangs from a pull-up bar
> Jumping goblet squats
> Kettlebell swings
> Suitcase carries
> Turkish getups

The recipient knew the kettlebell world well enough to make it work. As I look at this now, I'm a little surprised to see not only the whole family of fundamental human movements but also an excellent example of level changes. In case you need a "do this" workout, well: **Do this**.

## A Level Change Template

**Half-Kneeling Press**
**Hangs from a Pull Up Bar**
**Jumping Goblet Squats**
**Kettlebell Swings**
**Suitcase Carries**
**Turkish Get Ups**

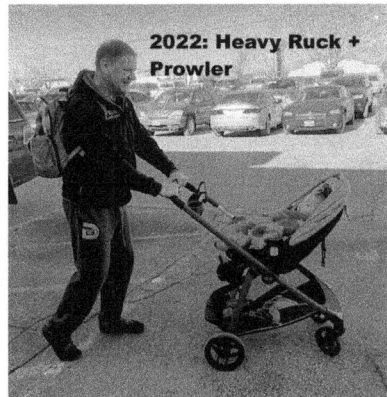

2022: Heavy Ruck + Prowler

This workout program reflects years of insight, hard work, and excellent feedback. I noted this a few years ago while still formulating this concept. Here are my notes:

*Training a "normal" person will be much easier. The "thinking" must be discussed first. The word "fractals" comes to mind: A fractal is a never-ending pattern. Fractal patterns are already familiar since nature is full of fractals: trees, rivers, coastlines, mountains, clouds, seashells, and hurricanes. A leaf looks like a tree and a small stone resembles a mountain. If done correctly, a training day can look like a career.*

*Jurassic Park discusses this same insight from another perspective:*

*"And that's how things are. A day is like a whole life. You start out doing one thing but end up doing something else. You plan to run an errand but never get there. . . . And at the end of your life, your whole existence has the same haphazard quality too. Your whole life has the same shape as a single day." Michael Crichton*

I have a simple model for training most people:

It's life.

This is a training program based on our movement history:

> We start off rolling around and crawling.
> Then, we get up on one knee.
> Then, back to the ground.
> We finally rise up and go after it for a while.
> We stumble and get back up.
> We stumble again and lie back down.
> And stay there!

This is also an excellent template for training.

> Naked Turkish getups (no weight) and ground-based mobility work
> Half-kneeling presses (alternate the knees down)—a few reps with both hands
> Bird dogs

Humane burpee or variation
Mobility movements from six-point position and half-kneeling
Naked Turkish getups
Easy foam rolling or correctives

The goal of this session is to "get sweaty" and build some strength, but most importantly, to leave the gym feeling better than when you arrived.

This training session can be expanded or contracted as appropriate.

**Most importantly, to leave the gym feeling better than when you arrived.**

None of this is new. Some of the basic level changes will be obvious to anyone who follows Tim Anderson's work:

On your back to prone: "Rolling"
Half-kneeling to on your back: "Shoulder roll"
Bear crawl: "Bear gait"

I'm only tasting the depths of Tim's work here, but his Pressing RESET method is based on how babies move from rolling to sprinting. You'll see this tying into his insights.

The humane burpee is a study of level changes. Remember, if you want to make it harder, just slide the goblet squats and pushups to 10. 10–9–8–7–6–5–4–3–2–1 gives you 55 total reps of the squat and pushup—and that's plenty of work for a single day, and in many cases, too much. If you're doing 10 swings, that's 100; if you choose 15 per round, it's 150.

That's "enough."

# Some Basic Level Training Combos

**Tim Anderson's Original Strength**

On your Back to Prone:
    "Rolling"

Half Kneeling to On your Back:
    "Shoulder Roll"

Bear "Gait":
    Bear Crawl

Humane Burpee (Dan Martin)

Swing/GS/Push Up

**Bear/Bear:**
    Bear Crawl-Bear Hug Carry

GS/Monkey Bar/Bear Crawl

GS/Prowler/Push Up

DL/Bear Crawl/Sprint

Hinge/Squat to Sprint
    "GS" is Goblet Squat

Another fun combination is the bear/bear, where we combine bear crawls with bear-hug carries. Working with a partner is illuminating as you'll quickly discover that both exercises are cardiovascular challenges.

One of our javelin throwers invented a very interesting training combination. The sector had been moved a little, so the run-up was next to a set of monkey bars. He came up with this combination:

    Goblet squat for eight reps
    Monkey bars
    Bear crawl for about 20 meters

It combined mobility, flexibility, hard breathing, and most of the training needed for this level of athlete. Moreover, it was "fun."

And...that season, we didn't have a SINGLE injury in our javelin crew. Monkey bar work is amazing for the health of javelin throwers. (If it isn't clear, javelin throwers tend to get more injuries than most throwers.)

For a large University American football team, I designed a little test for their indoor preseason training (and measurements):

> Five deadlift reps
> Bear crawl 10 yards
> Sprint 20 yards

Finally, the whole family of lift-n-sprints completely changed my career.

Remember: Strive to have nearly no time gap between the two movements. Go, go, go!

> The basics:
> Eight goblet squats followed immediately by a hard sprint (40–100 meters)

> My favorite:
> Eight overhead squats followed by a hard sprint

> *Go heavy on this one:*
> Kettlebell or barbell front squats followed by a hard sprint
> Certainly, add hills or sleds as appropriate and let your imagination run.

One small thing—and this is something we learned from hard experience: Just do three total lift-n-sprints. If you feel you should or could have done more, increase the load or intensity next time.

This workout focuses on quality, NOT quantity.

Unfortunately, few trainers and coaches (and lifters and clients) remember that quality training is the master key.

And this stuns many of us: what do we do now?

The great question then arises: well, I got hundreds of tools (machines, bells, chains, elastic bands, and variations of each) and a heavenly host of exercises from literally every place on the earth (Australian pushups, Romanian deadlifts, and Bulgarian Split Squats just to start), so what do I do?

Well, what do you have (equipment), what do you know (exercise selection), and what is the goal? In other words, what are your givens? It's time to think about geometry!

## The Geometry of Strength Training

*"Let no one ignorant of geometry enter."*

Tradition tells us this was on the door of Plato's Academy, his school in Athens. "Plato," by the way, was his nickname, meaning EITHER "broad shoulders" or "broad forehead". Of course, lifters should think it was his broad shoulders. No matter what, geometry remains the foundation of logic, philosophy, theology, and…weightlifting.

Geometry was the easiest class I took in high school. The study of shapes (and points and lines and planes) and the logic of doing proofs seemed so clear to me. I had some marvelous teachers in biology (Bob Jacobs) and physical education (indeed the whole staff), and I was destined to go in that direction. However, my math teacher, Robert Sawtell, saw my strengths in geometry class and challenged me to always do TWO proofs for each homework assignment and test question.

I am not bragging. Through my nearly fifty years as a coach and sixty years as a lifter, I have bumped into this interesting phenomenon over and over: the BEST coaches are firmly fixed on logic, in math (at some level), and on understanding the key to great coaching:

The Givens.

In geometry, the givens are the facts one builds upon. For example, Triangle ABC is a right triangle. This is one of the givens of this proof. Speaking of right triangles, it might surprise you that Pythagoras, our friend who taught us that $A^2 + B^2 = C^2$, was also the father-in-law and perhaps the coach of Milo of Croton, our first superstar in wrestling.

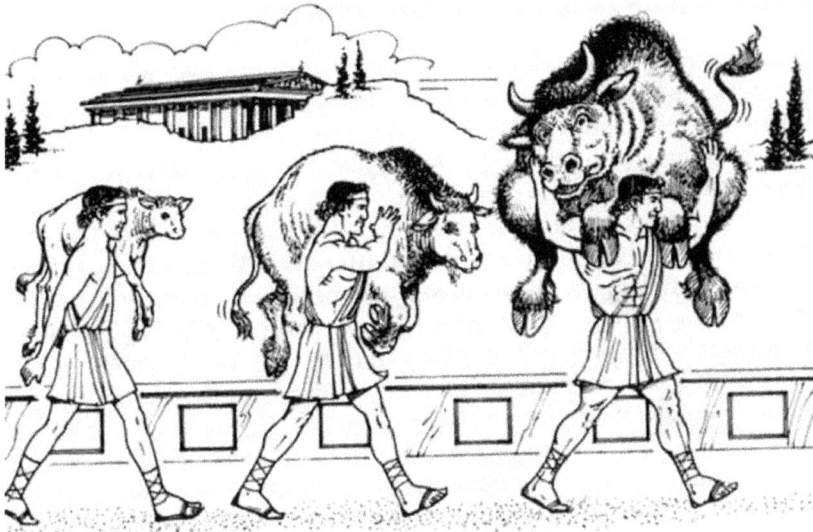

*Milo of Croton taught us the three basic principles of building muscle. Public Domain*

Milo consumed, we are told, a daily amount of twenty pounds of meat, twenty pounds of bread, and eighteen pints of wine. But that is not why we remember Milo. It was his idea to pick up a bull. Milo is the father of Progressive Resistance Exercise, and it's his fault that many people think that success in strength training is a straight line. I have joked many times with new lifters that if you bench 100 pounds today and only add ten pounds a week, about a year from now, you will bench over 600 pounds. It sure works on paper.

Remember: he CARRIED the bull. He didn't do skull crushers or curls with it.

Back to the Givens. Let me explain this with an example. Years ago, I did a workshop at a famous Big Ten football program. The new head coach was desperately trying to upgrade the facilities. The area was enormous and filled with every weight, plate, machine, toy, and equipment idea ever invented. There were also areas for food and drink throughout. An entire game, from American football to rugby in all its variations, could easily have been played in this facility.

Trying to mimic the training of this program would probably be impossible for every reader. Most coaches have a different set of "Givens."

Typical weight room givens:

> A few barbells (and some are still straight)
> A mishmash of weights and plates that rarely match
> Some broken machines, a lot of broken dumbbells, and medicine balls with holes
> A smell

Trying to adapt MY gym to do the workouts at this Big Ten school would be improbable at best. I coached a track and field program with these Givens:

> No track
> No field

I should also mention "no support," but, well, *that's a Given!*

The geometry of success is built on a key principle: you MUST accept and overcome your Givens. As we walk through this single example of Olympic lifting, I want you to understand the power of thinking. I firmly believe that thinking separates the great from the good, the good from the bad. (And the bad from the crap)

Basically, my simplified thought process for any coaching problem is a three-fold approach. This works for life, too:

# Asymmetrical Risks

What's the worst that can happen?

# Embrace the Obvious

What's the obvious solution?

# Respect the Process

Oddly, Little and Often over the Long Haul worked!

As I was writing this, the news shared a story of a young man who drowned in a local lake. He was paddleboarding without a life vest. The greatest asymmetrical risk for any watersport would be drowning. When I think: "What's the worst that can happen?"

*I would pop on my life vest.*

At my age, the most dangerous thing in the home is the floor. Falling causes an unusually high number of deaths after 60. So, I always take extra care getting in and out of the shower, and I keep the stairs clean and well-lit. You know the drill: buckle up, wear a helmet, check the blind spots when changing lanes, and look before you leap.

As a coach, I welcome the discussion before the game about this point: "What happens if we lose?" Sometimes, like when trying to get into the playoffs, we can discuss the next route to the championship. I often consider what will happen if my athletes have a bad day. These few seconds of thought often prepare me for the conversation after the competition.

After a good day, I will often tell an athlete what I would tell her if this would have been a BAD day. Oh…we laugh. But a moment of prep is far better than the agony of "winging it."

Embracing the obvious is probably something that is, well, obvious. My coaching message of "Throwers throw, jumpers jump, lifters lift, sprinters sprint" brings laughs at workshops.

Please laugh. Then, go to a typical training session. Throwers are running and jumping and, just at the end of the practice, maybe get a few throws. Online, sprint coaches argue to death the value of all kinds of things, while the best coaches focus on sprinting.

If you fear falling, practice some falling and install some safety bars. Obviously. If you fear financial issues, do what I learned half a century ago:

> Keep an emergency fund with easy access.
> Strive to remain in (or return to) debt-free status.
> Save for some future "thing."

I always joke that "Future Danny" will be so happy I saved this money for…whatever. My answer to most of life's and ALL coaching questions is "Embrace the Obvious."

Finally, one last boring truth: embrace the obvious, do it, and respect the process. Coach Ralph Maughan told me the secret to elite performance and almost all questions of life, with the phrase:

Little and often over the long haul.

What's better: flossing twice a day for a few months or having the dental hygienist take out some high-powered torture device to scrape the tartar off your teeth? What's better: saving for retirement starting at 18 or trying to win the lottery at 65?

As I tell my clients, you know the answer. There are no real secrets to success. So, save now, walk daily, sleep well, and drink water.

There are no secrets. The Geometry of Success is based on this truth.

I want to tell you the story of Dave Turner and the Hercules Bar Bell Club (HBBC). Dave was a geometry teacher and a life-long lover of the Olympic lifts. He took an abandoned closet next to the auditorium at his school and transformed it into a workable, although tight, training facility. Let me share my story with Dave from my book *Forty Years with a Whistle*.

## Dave Turner
*From Forty Years with a Whistle*

The Fall of 1980 was, well, "a time in my life." As I look back, it is a whirl of good and bad. My mother was strangely quiet about her cancer treatments, and I began full-time work on my Masters in history.

I continued to help the throwers at Utah State while being the "strength coach." Some athletes followed my advice and ideas, but many chose to skip lifting or train like bodybuilders. Their path did NOT lead to superlative performance. I had learned a lot in the year after graduating from college: I had worked in a cheese factory on the night shift (10 pm to 6:30 am) and juggled coaching, a few classes, and full-time work.

The one thing I didn't do much was sleep. I learned to "do without sleep!"

With a stipend from the University to study and a few work opportunities ("Assistant Director of the Utah History Fair"), the fall of 1980 promised to be a bit more normal. I was excited to sleep at night again rather than clean melted cheese off stainless-steel hoods, and I would be able to train again.

I got some news: the first Utah State Weightlifting Championship would be held in Salt Lake City a few months later. I started training again, and I contacted Dick Notmeyer, and he agreed to review my workouts. I started sending him weekly letters about my training, and he would reply with ideas and insights.

My training was going well. Then, I got a call at 3 am: "Mom just died." On October 2, 1980, my mother, Aileen Barbara McCloskey John, died after a rather quick battle with breast cancer.

Travel. Funeral. Sadness.

About three weeks later, twenty people descended on somewhere in the west side of Salt Lake City for the state weightlifting meet. It was at this time that I met the organizer, Dave Turner.

Dave deserves to be in multiple Hall of Fames, but I doubt he will get in. He single-handedly built Utah Olympic lifting. For decades, he ran meets, judged, lifted, organized, and coached O lifters. He was also a middle school math teacher who also developed a team called the "Hercules Bar Bell Club."

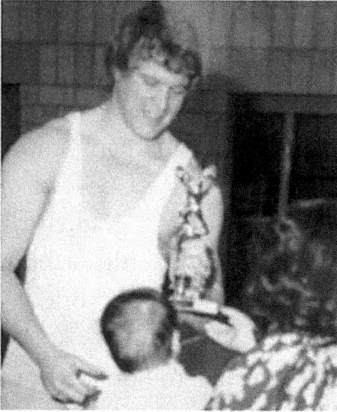

I'm still proud to be a member. In this picture is me being awarded Best Lifter at the State Meet in 1980. That's good, but what is truly interesting is the rest of the picture. See that baby? That baby's sons have lifted with me as fellow HBBC teammates. As I write this, the youngest organizes our state's Olympic lifting schedule.

Dave coached his team three days a week in a working closet just off the school's auditorium. The walls were filled with motivational pictures and the simple programs that Dave used to teach the lifts.

I always warn my interns and friends when they train with Dave: it will be a hard hour.

Wait, an hour? Yes, we start at 3:00 and go until 4:00.

Exactly.

Dave begins with a short meeting reminding the team about upcoming events and the usual details of performance sports: fill out the form, send the check, and show up.

Dave then has the team go through a full body flexibility warm-up that is a series of classic movements done one after another.

Dave's beginners use a simple program to learn and develop their rudiments of strength. After the general work, we do a ten-minute warm-up of shoulder "dislocates" with broomsticks, overhead squats with broomsticks, followed by front squats, then a "cardio-like" few minutes of snatches and clean and jerks with the broomsticks. Dave reinforces the terms used in lifting: "Get set," "Push the floor," "Jump," "Dip," and "Down."

Once, and Parker J. Burns was with me doing this, so we have Third Party verification on this; we went for twenty minutes. It was exhausting.

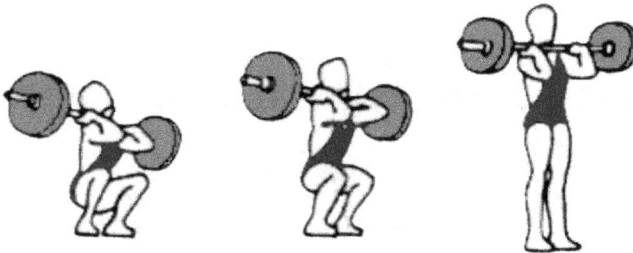

Then, we do Dave's daily program:

- Snatch: 8 Sets of Doubles (a "double" is two perfect repetitions)
- Clean and Jerk: 8 Sets of Singles (a "single" is a perfect repetition)
- Front Squat: 5 Sets of 5 Repetitions
- Press: 5 Sets of 3 Repetitions

If your form is perfect, you add weight the next workout; if not, you stay at the current weight. I know, I know, it looks easy on paper. Try it…then tell me it is easy.

After reviewing this after forty years of experience, I realize Dave is teaching his lifters how to lift during the warmups! I stole this idea for my discus throwers, and our throwers warm up with the basic movements…over and over and over again…of "Stretch-1-2-3." They hear the terms, do the movements and warm up their bodies and techniques simultaneously.

The genius of Dave's system is two-fold; first, the athletes prepare from the moment they enter the gym to lift on the platform at a meet. All their training is focused on the two meet lifts: the Snatch and the Clean and Jerk. The Front Squats and the Presses are the "strength" moves.

Then, at 3:58 or so, we clean up the weights, put our hands together, and shout the motto of the Olympic Games:

"Citius, Altius, Fortius!" (Latin for "Faster, Higher, Stronger")

Dave then walks us through our HBBC lifting contract:

## The Hercules Barbell Club Standards of Behavior

1. Club Oath: I will use my newfound strength for doing good as I abide by the four L's of life: LIVE, LOVE, LEARN, LIFT.
2. Club Motto: CITIUS, ALTIUS, FORTIUS.
3. Club Slogan: I will strive to follow the six D's of success: DREAM, DESIRE, DECISION, DISCIPLINE, DEDICATION, DETERMINATION.
4. Club Law: I will treat all people with respect, especially my teammates.

I've had a hard time driving home after these one-hour workouts.

Dave coached me in my 20s, 30s, 40s, 50s, and 60s. No, I don't lift like I did in my 30s, but I still lift. I appreciate his friendship, his coaching, and his genius.

Dave reinforced a "truth:" If you are going to perform, you MUST practice like you perform. Dave's template of getting everything done in one hour became my model for coaching track and field and, later, all my coaching opportunities (within reason).

Dave also has an advanced program for peaking at larger meets. This is the ten-week template:

|  | Day | One | Day | Two | Day Three |
|---|---|---|---|---|---|
| Week | Press | F Squat | Pull | F Squat | Total |
| 1 | 60/3/5 | 72/2/5 | 80/2/5 | 72/3/5 | 80 |
| 2 | 64/3/5 | 72/2/5 | 84/2/3 | 72/4/5 | 68 |
| 3 | 68/3/5 | 72/2/5 | 88/2/2 | 72/5/6 | 84 |
| 4 | 72/3/5 | 72/2/5 | 92/1/2 | 76/5/5 | 72 |
| 5 | 76/2/4 | 72/2/5 | 96/1/2 | 80/4/4 | 88 |
| 6 | 80/2/3 | 72/2/5 | 100/1/1 | 84/3/3 | 76 |
| 7 | 84/2/2 | 72/2/5 | 104/1/1 | 88/2/2 | 92 |
| 8 | 88/1/1 | 72/2/5 | 108/1/1 | 104/1/1 | 80 |
| 9 | Total 76 |  | Total 80 |  | 84 |
| 10 | Total 76 |  | Rest |  | Meet 100+ |

Day One
Press: Push Jerks or Jerks
F Squat: Front Squats

Day Two
Pull: Snatch Grip High Pulls and Clean Grip High Pulls
F Squat: Front Squats

<u>Day Three and Last Two Weeks</u>
Total: Practice as if this is an Olympic lifting meet. (I found that doing a long workout helped; full warm up. Snatch up to "opener" then make three lifts perfectly. Repeat for Clean and Jerk)

The numbers: the first number is the percent, the second is the reps, and the third is the number of sets.

I recommend the full warm-up and stick work, too.

Dave gave me a program in 2010 that culminated all his years of experience. He told me, "I had you in mind" for this program.

## Hercules Bar Bell Club Rack Routine

<u>Day One</u>
Snatch: 80% for three singles
Low Front Squat Isometric: 100% for a Six Second Hold in the Rack
High Snatch Pull Isometric: 100% for a Six Second Hold in the Rack
Push Press: 60% for three sets of two

<u>Day Two</u>
Clean and Jerk: 80% for three singles
Mid Clean Pull Isometric: Two x 100% for a Six Second Hold in the Rack
High Front Squat: Two x 100% for a Six Second Hold in the Rack
Lockout: 100% for a Six Second Hold in the Rack

<u>Day Three</u>
Total with at least 80%. Meet conditions.

On Week Eight, test or compete.
Monday: Total with 76 %
Rest all week.
Meet: Go for Records.

Again, do the full warm-up and broomstick work daily.

So, not long after burying my mother, I lifted in the first Utah State Weightlifting Championships. I was awarded "Best Lifter" and competed in the championships numerous times since then. I've lifted with Dave Turner in gyms, correctional facilities, fire stations, and garages. I competed alongside him, his sons, and his grandsons, representing Hercules BBC.

Dave kept me competing until I had the spark to step it back up again.

I honor our friendship.

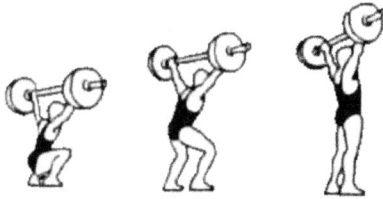

## Adapting the Dave Turner Program

I have made a few changes to my training as I approach age 70, and recommend it to those who want to be "Fit to Lift." When I was in high school, we used to get a magazine from school called "Conditioning for a Purpose." The United States Army sponsored it and, in hindsight, was excellent. The idea of "a purpose" has stuck with me for over fifty years.

**The idea of "a purpose" has stuck with me for over fifty years.**

I break up my thrower's training into two basic yearly goals:

Fit goes far.
Smooth goes far
(And thank you to the late John Powell for instilling this in me)

To get fit for a specific task, or "condition for a purpose," isn't the same as just joining a gym and hoping for the best. My adaption of Dave's program gets me ready to lift in meets, drop body fat, and still lift and live long past my "official" retirement.

When I revisited the HBBC program, I made the same mistakes I made in the 1960s, 1970s, 1980s, 1990s, 2000s, 2010s, and 2020s… and beyond!!!

I went way too heavy.

Can I do twenty-six sets of Olympic lifts and strength movements? Well, yes, certainly!

In thirty to forty minutes…well…hmmm…maybe? So, we must adjust the load.

Making it as simple as possible, pressing 30 kilos for 15 reps, snatching 40 for 16 reps, clean and jerking 50 for 8, reps and squatting 60 for 25 total reps looks easy on paper. However, cramming it all into a tight window of time changes everything.

I chose relatively light loads in this example. Simply bumping up to 50 kilos on the press, 60 on the snatches, 70 on the clean and jerk, and 80 on the front squat Is a serious and hard workout…considering the time restrictions.

I never understood why Dave had the athletes do this until I did it. If you have the courage to train on task like this three days a week for a while, you will be rewarded with some serious conditioning. Then, when a meet appears on the horizon, shift to one of Dave's peaking programs and prep for the platform.

Then, I came up with a "better" solution for getting fit for Olympic lifting meets: one bar and one load. Again, this is going to be easy on paper. I had to make one adjustment: I started with the clean and press first. So:

Warmups
Press 5 Sets of 3
Snatch: 8 Sets of Doubles
Clean and Jerk: 8 Sets of Singles
Front Squat: 5 Sets of 5

I see the clean and press as a warmup on this program.

So, how did I make this "even harder?" The sets start Every Minute On the Minute, or EMOM. I use an old clock with a sweeping second hand. When the hand hits "12," I go. The workout is 26 sets in 26 minutes, and I am sweating and heaving when I finish…regardless of load.

Since I squat clean every press and front squat, the number of squats is "more" than you initially think. One might also miss how the exercises "wave" a bit in intensity. I see the clean and press section and clean and jerk section as a bit easier than the snatch and squat portions. The snatches and squats really get my heart rate up, so we have a little bit of waving of the exercise intensity doing this order.

As a switch-up, especially if one needs more warmup and lubrication for the snatch, try this order occasionally:

Clean and Jerk
Front squat
Clean and press
Snatch

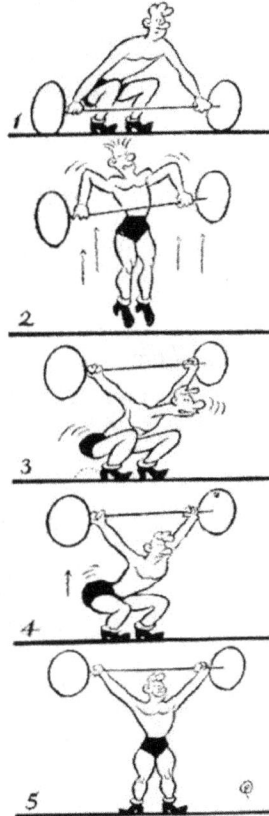

HOW TO DO THE SQUAT SNATCH

Those single clean and jerks are relatively easy and give me eight minutes to get greased up for the front squats. The press doesn't have a lot of big movements (just one squat clean), so I can regroup there before the snatches. The snatch seems to take a lot of energy no matter where I put the lift, so finishing with this lift leans into the classic idea of a finisher at the end of a workout.

Years ago, Mike Warren Brown wrote an online article about the importance of Mentors in training and coaching. He summed up my lessons from Dave like this:

> *The next point in Dan's coaching lineage is Dave Turner, whom he met in 1980. Dave leads the Hercules Barbell Club in Salt Lake City. From Dave, Dan took three major principles:*
>
> > *Accumulate your strength over years.*
> > *Get into condition for your sport by doing your sport.*
> > *Come in a little undertrained versus overtrained (It's true, but hard to believe)*

The third point was also echoed by legendary lifter and coach Tommy Kono in his book, Weightlifting, Olympic Style.

## The Index Card Idea

I don't know about you, Gentle Reader, but I struggle to keep track of sets in a workout. I start fiddling around with home repairs and chores, and wander off and come back, and I can't remember how many sets I did. With eight sets in the HBBC program, Dave showed me an idea years ago that I carried into my coaching, too.

Oddly, Dave doesn't remember telling me this!

It's simple: grab some note cards or whatever you have and write the lift, the reps and sets, and a number (one to eight for the eight sets). I keep mine in a Ziplock bag and pull all the cards out (Press, Snatch, Clean and Jerk, and Front Squat). After each set, I flip the card, read the quote, and recover...quickly. At the end of the workout, I slide all the cards in the bag for the next workout.

My snatch and clean and jerk cards look like this:

| Front | Back |
|-------|------|
| Snatch<br>8 sets of 2<br>One | "Joe Mills believes weightlifting should be a "way of life," aimed at teaching young men and women inner toughness, discipline, and concentration. |
| Snatch<br>8 sets of 2<br>Two | "As the workout proceeds, it becomes clear that in response to Mills' comments, all three lifters are quickly making adjustments which improves their lifts. Grillo, for example, brings his feet closer at the start of the pull and, as a result, finds he can use his quadriceps more effectively." |
| Snatch<br>8 sets of 2<br>Three | By doing the lifts three times a week, Brusie's developing the core muscles, all the little muscles you use for lifting. "To be good at lifting, you have to lift," says Mills. "Also, my lifters always know exactly what they are capable of lifting. In competition, they can start with ten pounds more than their best in training." |

| Front | Back |
|---|---|
| Snatch<br>8 sets of 2<br>Four | "You're stubbing your toe on the jerk. And your shoulders are dropping down as soon as the bar comes off the floor. You've got to keep them back." "Is that it?" Klonoski with some surprise. "I was told I was arm pulling, but that didn't sound right." "It wasn't right," retorts Mills. "Letting your shoulders drop slows you down." |
| Snatch<br>8 sets of 2<br>Five | "Say a guy is snatching 95kg.," Mills explains. "I'd have him start with 65kg. for five reps, 70 for five, 75 for 5, and then take single attempts in 2.5 kg. jumps to 90kg. That's 21 lifts. If he makes all 21, he adds 2.5kg. to all attempts in the snatch session. So he'd start with 67.5. If he misses the last lift (90kg.), he stays with the same 65 kg. starter, no increase. If he misses several of the heavier lifts, he is probably just tired. He should listen to his body and rest." |
| Snatch<br>8 sets of 2<br>Six | "Mills believes that the York courses, including the fast deadlifts and repetition squats, remain the best general conditioners for weightlifting." |

| Front | Back |
|---|---|
| Snatch<br>8 sets of 2<br>Seven | "You're feeling that weight. It should all be one movement. Look up at the top of the pull and jump down fast. All one movement. Time it right, and the weight will feel like it's pulling you up from the bottom position."<br>Joe Mills |
| Snatch<br>8 sets of 2<br>Eight | "But if I can get a lifter down to one mistake per lift, that's acceptable. With two or three, he won't lift to his potential."<br>Joe Mills |
| Clean and Jerk<br>8 sets of 1<br>One | "Don't think you're ill-equipped!"<br>Joe Mills |
| Clean and Jerk<br>8 sets of 1<br>Two | You're never as tired as you think you are!"<br>Joe Mills |
| Clean and Jerk<br>8 sets of 1<br>Three | "Better to be under-trained than over-trained."<br>Tommy Kono |
| Clean and Jerk<br>8 sets of 1<br>Four | "A good lifter…does not make excuses. Whatever you have, think that it could have been worse, so be grateful."<br>Tommy Kono |

| Front | Back |
|---|---|
| Clean and Jerk<br>8 sets of 1<br>Five | "With complacency comes eventual regression."<br>Tommy Kono |
| Clean and Jerk<br>8 sets of 1<br>Six | "For every "down" there should be an "up," but you can stay "down" if you tax yourself too often."<br>Tommy Kono |
| Clean and Jerk<br>8 sets of 1<br>Seven | "Training hard and lifting heavy are all important, but your belief in your own ability is what makes you a champion."<br>Tommy Kono |
| Clean and Jerk<br>8 sets of 1<br>Eight | "Think, plan, and expect positive results."<br>Tommy Kono |

After each set, I pick up the card and flip it over. I expanded the idea by putting little quotes and sayings on the back of the cards. Feel free to find your own quotes, but these tiny quotes inspire me.

**Note:** On my press and front squat cards, I include quick mobility and flexibility movements from Tim Anderson's Pressing RESET method.

Tim sent this email to me a few years ago after I decided to Olympic lift again after double total hip replacements:

*Morning Prep*

    A.  *Get in a six-point rock position, dorsiflexed on the balls of your feet, and push your hips back towards your feet as far as they will comfortably go while you maintain a silverback gorilla back, and nod your head up and down for 1 minute. Keep your tongue on the roof of your mouth. Lead the motion with your eyes. DO NOT move into pain anywhere...*

    B.  *Same position and look over your shoulder from left to right. You are rotating your head, trying to find your back pockets with your eyes. Let your spine follow your head. Do this for one minute. Keep your tongue on the roof of your mouth.*

    C.  *Rocking with feet dorsiflexed, on the balls of your feet x 2 minutes. Keep your head up, eyes on the horizon, tongue on the roof of your mouth. Don't lose your gorilla back.*

    D.  *The egg roll x 2 minutes.*

*Do this sequence every day. I want to give you more, but you asked for 3 to 4 movements, so I think we should start here. By the way, I am assuming you practice or live by diaphragmatic breathing. Oh, and let me know if you want one more movement.*

*<u>Do this In between and right before your Olympic Lift (snatch, clean and jerk, etc...)</u>*

*Ok, let's do something that is crazy enough to work. Before you snatch or clean, I'd like you to do a set of eight explosive rock-drops in the 6-point rocking position. I've thought up this just for you - but it will work. You will see...*

*What you do is this: you rock, BUT you slowly rock your weight over your hands, like your slow practice pull from the ground. Then, explosively push your butt back towards your feet (be fast) to the bottom of the rocking position depth you can achieve without losing a gorilla back, dropping your head, or moving into pain. Do this for eight reps between and around your OLY sets.*

*Thank you, Tim!!*

For most of us, the following are fine:

# Tim Anderson Pressing RESET Materials

*Thank you, Tim. Your contributions to the world of fitness are vastly underappreciated. You make a difference in this world.*

### Prone Neck Nods

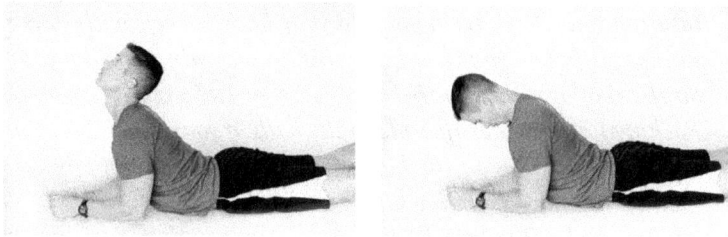

- Lie on your belly
- Prop up on your elbows
- Leading with your eyes, look up and nod your head up
- Look down and nod your head down

### Find Your Shoes

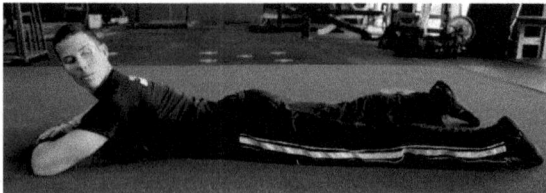

- Lie on your belly
- Prop up on your elbows
- Leading with your eyes, look left and rotate your head to the left
- Look right and rotate your head to the right
- Try to find your shoes

## Six-Point Nods

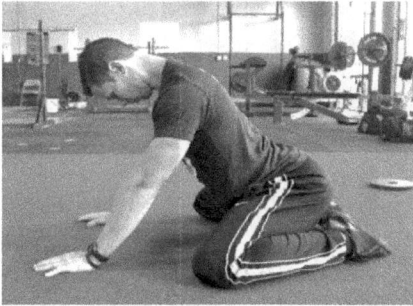

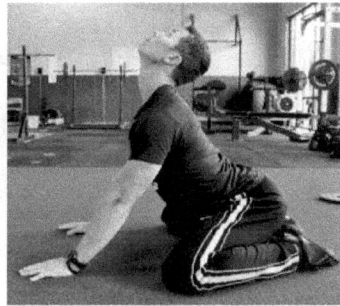

- Get on your hands and knees
- Keep a tall sternum (flat gorilla back)
- Leading with your eyes, look up and nod your head up
- Look down and nod your head down

## Six-Point Rocking

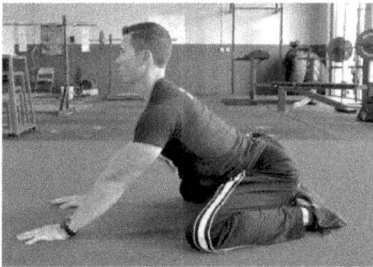

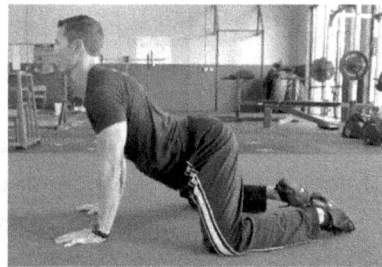

- Get on your hands and knees
- Keep a tall sternum (flat gorilla back)
- Keep your head UP on the horizon
- Rock back and forth as far as you can without losing your tall sternum and without dropping your head.

## Grizzly Bear Crawl

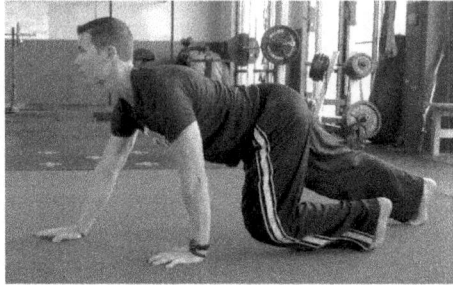

- Crawl on your hands and feet
- Keep your head up on the horizon
- Keep a tall sternum (flat gorilla back)
- Keep your butt down below your head—back level with the ground
- Move opposite limbs together

## Cross-Crawl

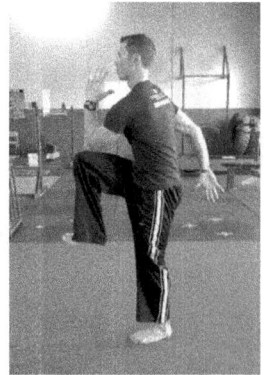

- Stand tall
- Touch your opposite elbow to your opposite knee
- Alternate back and forth between sides
- If you cannot touch elbow to knee without bending over, touch the opposite hand to thigh.

From the ABCs (and Fs) to the Geometry of Strength, I have strived to teach you, gentle reader, that with a few minutes of mental effort, you can design a fabulous program with whatever tools, equipment, and goals you seek.

Not every exercise is necessary to achieve one's vision and one's goals. As I argue daily, ENOUGH is enough when it comes to sets, reps, loads, time periods, and exercise choices. Enough is also a good way to think of calories, but that is another discussion.

Using the ABCs (and Fs) to make some preliminary decisions and then branching out into level changes will quickly make you an indispensable cog in any gym, team, or training community. Dave Turner's example reminds us that we can all pardon the cliché from forty years ago, "Bloom where we are planted."

No matter how bad you think you have it, somebody else has it worse! And...sometimes, having the perfect facility and system impedes wonderful opportunities to invent some crazy exercise, device, or scheme that might change the world.

I'm looking at YOU goblet squat!

So, there you go. Now go...and do!

# Never Let Go!

# Learn More

## COACH DAN JOHN

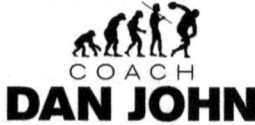

Dan John has been lifting since 1965 and has won national championships in the discus throw, Olympic lifting, Highland Games, and the Weight Pentathlon. He was recently awarded a Lifetime Achievement Award from Great Britain for his contributions to the field of strength and conditioning. A Fulbright Scholar, he has vast experience in scholarship, academics, and athletics. Dan has advanced degrees in history and religious education and has studied at the University of Haifa, the American University of Cairo, and Cornell. He is a former Senior Lecturer at Saint Mary's University in Twickenham, England.

His books include bestsellers such as Easy Strength Omnibook, Never Let Go, Mass Made Simple, and Intervention (among almost two dozen other published works) and countless articles. He is the grandfather to five and continues to write, coach, train, and lecture to practically every fitness and performance level.

His website is https://danjohnuniversity.com/

Enjoy his YouTube channel at
https://www.youtube.com/@DanJohnStrengthCoach

Find him on Instagram at https://www.instagram.com/coachdanjohn/